The Keto Chaffles Unmissable Recipes

An Unmissable Recipe Collection for Your Chaffles Meals

Kade Harrison

Table of Contents

Zucchini & Basil Chaffles

Servings: 2

Cooking Time:

10 Minutes

Ingredients:

- 1 organic egg, beaten
- ¼ cup Mozzarella cheese, shredded
- 2 tablespoons Parmesan cheese, grated
- ½ of small zucchini, grated and squeezed
- ¼ teaspoon dried basil, crushed
- Freshly ground black pepper, as required

Directions:

1. Preheat a mini waffle iron and then grease it.
2. In a medium bowl, place all ingredients and mix until well combined.
3. Place half of the mixture into preheated waffle iron and cook for about 4-5 minutes or until golden brown.
4. Repeat with the remaining mixture.

5. Serve warm.

Nutrition:

Calories: Net Carb: 1g Fat: 4.1g Saturated Fat: 1.7g
Carbohydrates: 1.3g Dietary Fiber: 0.3g Sugar: 0.7g
Protein: 6.1g

Hash Brown Chaffle

Servings: 2

Cooking Time:

10 Minutes

Ingredients:

- 1 large jicama root, peeled and shredded
- ½ medium onion, minced
- 2 garlic cloves, pressed
- 1 cup cheddar shredded cheese
- 2 eggs
- Salt and pepper, to taste

Directions:

1. Place jicama in a colander, sprinkle with 2 tsp salt, and let drain.
2. Squeeze out all excess liquid.
3. Microwave jicama for 5-8 minutes.
4. Mix ¾ of cheese and all other ingredients in a bowl.

5. Sprinkle 1-2 tsp cheese on waffle maker, add 3 Tbsp mixture, and top with 1-2 tsp cheese.
6. Cook for 5-minutes, or until done.
7. Remove and repeat for remaining batter.
8. Serve while hot with preferred toppings.

Nutrition:

Carbs: g ;Fat: 6 g ;Protein: 4 g ;Calories: 194

Breakfast Chaffle Sandwich

Servings: 1

Cooking Time:

10 Minutes

Ingredients:

- 2 basics cooked chaffles
- Cooking spray
- 2 slices bacon
- 1 egg

Directions:

1. Spray your pan with oil.
2. Place it over medium heat.
3. Cook the bacon until golden and crispy.
4. Put the bacon on top of one chaffle.
5. In the same pan, cook the egg without mixing until the yolk is set.
6. Add the egg on top of the bacon.
7. Top with another chaffle.

Nutrition:

Calories 514 Total Fat 47 g Saturated Fat 27 g
Cholesterol 274 mg Sodium 565 mg Potassium 106 mg
Total Carbohydrate 2 g Dietary Fiber 1 g Protein 21 g
Total Sugars 1 g

Cookie Dough Chaffle

Servings:4

Cooking Time:

7–9 Minutes

Ingredients:

- Batter
- 4 eggs
- ¼ cup heavy cream
- 1 teaspoon vanilla extract
- ¼ cup stevia
- 6 tablespoons coconut flour
- 1 teaspoon baking powder
- Pinch of salt
- ¼ cup unsweetened chocolate chips
- Other
- 2 tablespoons cooking spray to brush the waffle maker
- ¼ cup heavy cream, whipped

Directions:

1. Preheat the waffle maker.
2. Add the eggs and heavy cream to a bowl and stir in the vanilla extract, stevia, coconut flour, baking powder, and salt. Mix until just combined.
3. Stir in the chocolate chips and combine.
4. Brush the heated waffle maker with cooking spray and add a few tablespoons of the batter.
5. Close the lid and cook for about 7–8 minutes depending on your waffle maker.
6. Serve with whipped cream on top.

Nutrition:

Calories 3, fat 32.3 g, carbs 12.6 g, sugar 0.5 g, Protein 9 g, sodium 117 mg

Thanksgiving Pumpkin Spice Chaffle

Servings:4

Cooking Time:

5 minutes

Ingredients:

- 1 cup egg whites
- ¼ cup pumpkin puree
- 2 tsps. pumpkin pie spice
- 2 tsps. coconut flour
- ½ tsp. vanilla
- 1 tsp. baking powder
- 1 tsp. baking soda
- 1/8 tsp cinnamon powder
- 1 cup mozzarella cheese, grated
- 1/2 tsp. garlic powder

Directions:

1. Switch on your square waffle maker. Spray with non-stick spray.

2. Beat egg whites with beater, until fluffy and white.
3. Add pumpkin puree, pumpkin pie spice, coconut flour in egg whites and beat again.
4. Stir in the cheese, cinnamon powder, garlic powder, baking soda, and powder.
5. Pour ½ of the batter in the waffle maker.
6. Close the maker and cook for about 3 minutesutes.
7. Repeat with the remaining batter.
8. Remove chaffles from the maker.
9. Serve hot and enjoy!

Nutrition:

Protein: 51% 66 kcal Fat: 41% 53 kcal Carbohydrates: 8% kcal

Pumpkin Spice Chaffles

Servings: 2

Cooking Time:

14 Minutes

Ingredients:

- 1 egg, beaten
- ½ tsp pumpkin pie spice
- ½ cup finely grated mozzarella cheese
- 1 tbsp sugar-free pumpkin puree

Directions:

1. Preheat the waffle iron.
2. In a medium bowl, mix all the ingredients.
3. Open the iron, pour in half of the batter, close, and cook until crispy, 6 to 7 minutes.
4. Remove the chaffle onto a plate and set aside.
5. Make another chaffle with the remaining batter.
6. Allow cooling and serve afterward.

Nutrition Info:

Calories 90 Fats 6.46g Carbs 1.98g Net Carbs 1.58g
Protein 5.94g

Chaffle Fruit Snacks

Servings: 2

Cooking Time:

14 Minutes

Ingredients:

- 1 egg, beaten
- ½ cup finely grated cheddar cheese
- ½ cup Greek yogurt for topping
- 8 raspberries and blackberries for topping

Directions:

1. Preheat the waffle iron.
2. Mix the egg and cheddar cheese in a medium bowl.
3. Open the iron and add half of the mixture. Close and cook until crispy, 7 minutes.
4. Remove the chaffle onto a plate and make another with the remaining mixture.
5. Cut each chaffle into wedges and arrange on a plate.

6. Top each waffle with a tablespoon of yogurt and then two berries.
7. Serve afterward.

Nutrition:

Calories 207 Fats 15.29g Carbs 4.36g Net Carbs 3g Protein 12.91g

Open-faced Ham & Green Bell Pepper Chaffle Sandwich

Servings: 2

Cooking Time:

10 Minutes

Ingredients:

- 2 slices ham
- Cooking spray
- 1 green bell pepper, sliced into strips
- 2 slices cheese
- 1 tablespoon black olives, pitted and sliced
- 2 basic chaffles

Directions:

1. Cook the ham in a pan coated with oil over medium heat.
2. Next, cook the bell pepper.
3. Assemble the open-faced sandwich by topping each chaffle with ham and cheese, bell pepper and olives.

4. Toast in the oven until the cheese has melted a little.

Nutrition:

Calories 36 Total Fat 24.6g Saturated Fat 13.6g
Cholesterol 91mg Sodium 1154mg Potassium 440mg
Total Carbohydrate 8g Dietary Fiber 2.6g Protein 24.5g
Total Sugars 6.3g

Taco Chaffle

Servings: 4

Cooking Time:

20 Minutes

Ingredients:

- 1 tablespoon olive oil
- 1 lb. ground beef
- 1 teaspoon ground cumin
- 1 teaspoon chili powder
- ¼ teaspoon onion powder
- ½ teaspoon garlic powder
- Salt to taste
- 4 basic chaffles
- 1 cup cabbage, chopped
- 4 tablespoons salsa (sugar-free)

Directions:

1. Pour the olive oil into a pan over medium heat.
2. Add the ground beef.

3. Season with the salt and spices.

4. Cook until brown and crumbly.

5. Fold the chaffle to create a "taco shell".

6. Stuff each chaffle taco with cabbage.

7. Top with the ground beef and salsa.

Nutrition:

Calories 255 Total Fat 10.9g Saturated Fat 3.2g
Cholesterol 101mg Sodium 220mg Potassium 561mg
Total Carbohydrate 3g Dietary Fiber 1g Protein 35.1g
Total Sugars 1.3g

Christmas Morning Choco Chaffle Cake

Servings:8

Cooking Time:

5 minutes

Ingredients:

- 8 keto chocolate square chaffles
- 2 cups peanut butter
- 16 oz. raspberries

Directions:

1. Assemble chaffles in layers.
2. Spread peanut butter in each layer.
3. Top with raspberries.
4. Enjoy cake on Christmas morning with keto coffee!

Nutrition:

Protein: 3% 1Kcal Fat: 94% 207 Kcal Carbohydrates: 3% 15 Kcal

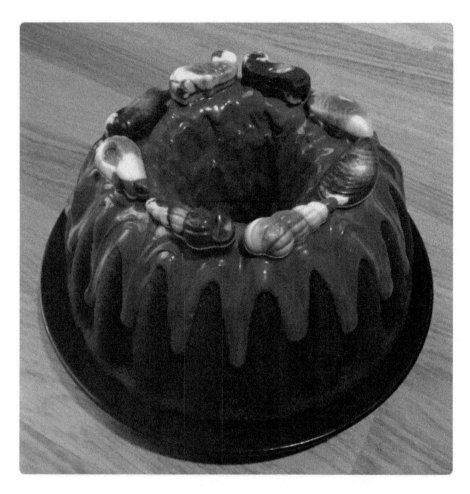

Lt Chaffle Sandwich

Servings: 2

Cooking Time:

15 Minutes

Ingredients:

- Cooking spray
- 4 slices bacon
- 1 tablespoon mayonnaise
- 4 basic chaffles
- 2 lettuce leaves
- 2 tomato slices

Directions:

1. Coat your pan with foil and place it over medium heat.
2. Cook the bacon until golden and crispy.
3. Spread mayo on top of the chaffle.
4. Top with the lettuce, bacon and tomato.
5. Top with another chaffle.

Nutrition:

Calories 238 Total Fat 18.4g Saturated Fat 5.
Cholesterol 44mg Sodium 931mg Potassium 258mg
Total Carbohydrate 3g Dietary Fiber 0.2g Protein 14.3g
Total Sugars 0.9g

Mozzarella Peanut Butter Chaffle

Servings: 2

Cooking Time:

15 Minutes

Ingredients:

- 1 egg, lightly beaten
- 2 tbsp peanut butter
- 2 tbsp Swerve
- 1/2 cup mozzarella cheese, shredded

Directions:

1. Preheat your waffle maker.
2. In a bowl, mix egg, cheese, Swerve, and peanut butter until well combined.
3. Spray waffle maker with cooking spray.
4. Pour half batter in the hot waffle maker and cook for minutes or until golden brown. Repeat with the remaining batter.
5. Serve and enjoy.

Nutrition:

Calories 150 Fat 11.5 g Carbohydrates 5g Sugar 1.7 g
Protein 8.8 g Cholesterol 86 mg

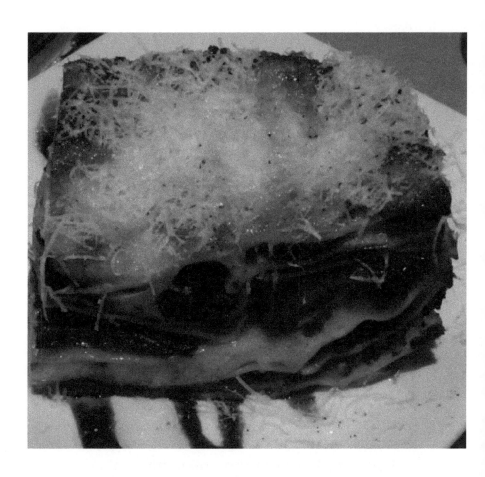

Double Decker Chaffle

Servings:2

Cooking Time:

10 Minutes

Ingredients:

- 1 large egg
- 1 cup shredded cheese
- TOPPING
- 1 keto chocolate ball
- 2 oz. cranberries
- 2 oz. blueberries
- 4 oz. cranberries puree

Directions:

1. Make 2 minutes dash waffles.
2. Put cranberries and blueberries in the freezer for about hours.
3. For serving, arrange keto chocolate ball between 2 chaffles.
4. Top with frozen berries,

5. Serve and enjoy!

Nutrition:

Protein: 23% 78 kcal Fat: % 223 kcal Carbohydrates: 9% 31 kcal

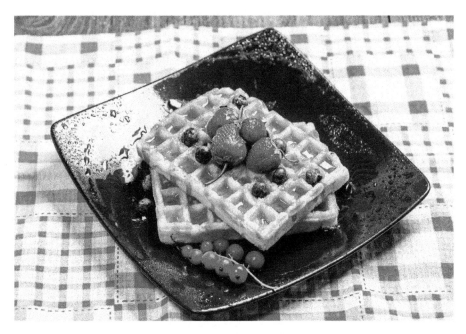

Cinnamon And Vanilla Chaffle

Servings: 4

Cooking Time:

7–9 Minutes

Ingredients:

- Batter
- 4 eggs
- 4 ounces sour cream
- 1 teaspoon vanilla extract
- 1 teaspoon cinnamon
- ¼ cup stevia
- 5 tablespoons coconut flour
- Other
- 2 tablespoons coconut oil to brush the waffle maker
- ½ teaspoon cinnamon for garnishing the chaffles

Directions:

1. Preheat the waffle maker.

2. Add the eggs and sour cream to a bowl and stir with a wire whisk until just combined.
3. Add the vanilla extract, cinnamon, and stevia and mix until combined.
4. Stir in the coconut flour and stir until combined.
5. Brush the heated waffle maker with coconut oil and add a few tablespoons of the batter.
6. Close the lid and cook for about 7–8 minutes depending on your waffle maker.
7. Serve and enjoy.

Nutrition:

Calories 224, fat 11 g, carbs 8.4 g, sugar 0.5 g, Protein 7.7 g, sodium 77 mg

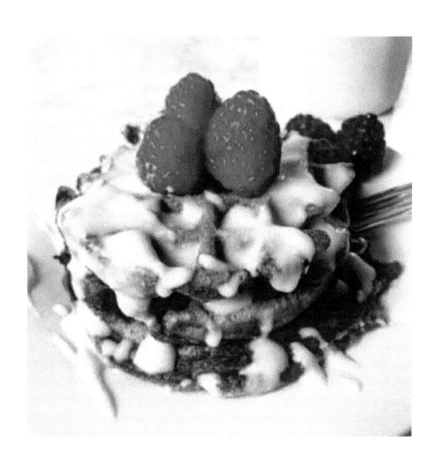

New Year Cinnamon Chaffle With Coconut Cream

Servings:2

Cooking Time:

5 minutes

Ingredients:

- 2 large eggs
- 1/8 cup almond flour
- 1 tsp. cinnamon powder
- 1 tsp. sea salt
- 1/2 tsp. baking soda
- 1 cup shredded mozzarella
- FOR TOPPING
- 2 tbsps. coconut cream
- 1 tbsp. unsweetened chocolate sauce

Directions:

1. Preheat waffle maker according to the manufacturer's directions.

2. Mix together recipe ingredients in a mixing bowl.
3. Add cheese and mix well.
4. Pour about ½ cup mixture into the center of the waffle maker and cook for about 2-3 minutesutes until golden and crispy.
5. Repeat with the remaining batter.
6. For serving, coat coconut cream over chaffles. Drizzle chocolate sauce over chaffle.
7. Freeze chaffle in the freezer for about10 minutesutes.
8. Serve on Christmas morning and enjoy!

Nutrition:

Protein: 3 100 kcal Fat: 56% 145 kcal Carbohydrates: 5% 13 kcal

Chaffles And Ice-cream Platter

Servings: 2

Cooking Time:

5 minutes

Ingredients:

- 2 keto brownie chaffles
- 2 scoop vanilla keto ice cream
- 8 oz. strawberries, sliced
- keto chocolate sauce

Directions:

1. Arrange chaffles, ice-cream, strawberries slice in serving plate.
2. Drizzle chocolate sauce on top.
3. Serve and enjoy!

Nutrition:

Protein: 26% kcal Fat: 68% 128 kcal Carbohydrates: 6% 11 kcal

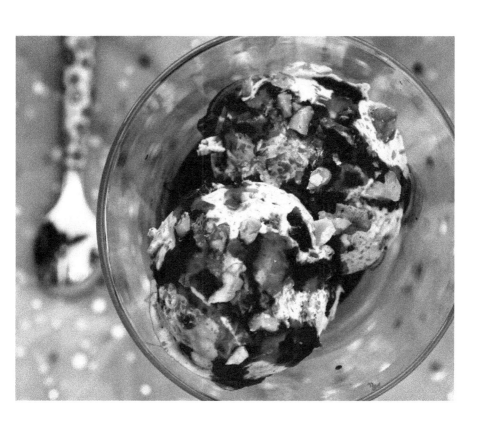

Choco Chip Pumpkin Chaffle

Servings: 2

Cooking Time:

15 Minutes

Ingredients:

- 1 egg, lightly beaten
- 1 tbsp almond flour
- 1 tbsp unsweetened chocolate chips
- 1/4 tsp pumpkin pie spice
- 2 tbsp Swerve
- 1 tbsp pumpkin puree
- 1/2 cup mozzarella cheese, shredded

Directions:

1. Preheat your waffle maker.
2. In a small bowl, mix egg and pumpkin puree.
3. Add pumpkin pie spice, Swerve, almond flour, and cheese and mix well.
4. Stir in chocolate chips.
5. Spray waffle maker with cooking spray.

6. Pour half batter in the hot waffle maker and cook for 4 minutes. Repeat with the remaining batter.
7. Serve and enjoy.

Nutrition:

Calories 130Fat 9.2 g Carbohydrates 5.9 g Sugar 0.6 g Protein 6.6 g Cholesterol mg

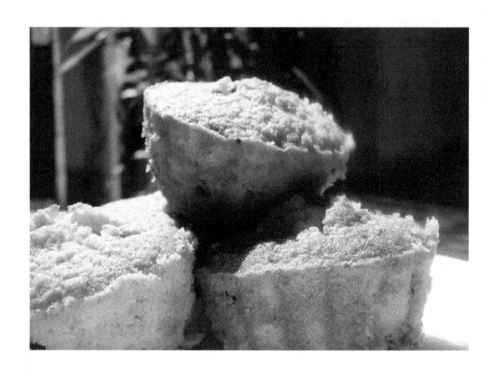

Sausage & Pepperoni Chaffle Sandwich

Servings: 4

Cooking Time:

10 Minutes

Ingredients:

- Cooking spray
- 2 cervelat sausage, sliced into rounds
- 12 pieces pepperoni
- 6 mushroom slices
- 4 teaspoons mayonnaise
- 4 big white onion rings
- 4 basic chaffles

Directions:

1. Spray your skillet with oil.
2. Place over medium heat.
3. Cook the sausage until brown on both sides.
4. Transfer on a plate.

5. Cook the pepperoni and mushrooms for 2 minutes.
6. Spread mayo on top of the chaffle.
7. Top with the sausage, pepperoni, mushrooms and onion rings.
8. Top with another chaffle.

Nutrition:

Calories 373 Total Fat 24.4g Saturated Fat 6g
Cholesterol 27mg Sodium 717mg Potassium 105mg
Total Carbohydrate 28g Dietary Fiber 1.1g Protein 8.1g
Total Sugars 4.5g

Pizza Flavored Chaffle

Servings: 3

Cooking Time:

12 Minutes

Ingredients:

- 1 egg, beaten
- ½ cup cheddar cheese, shredded
- 2 tablespoons pepperoni, chopped
- 1 tablespoon keto marinara sauce
- 4 tablespoons almond flour
- 1 teaspoon baking powder
- ½ teaspoon dried Italian seasoning
- Parmesan cheese, grated

Directions:

1. Preheat your waffle maker.
2. In a bowl, mix the egg, cheddar cheese, pepperoni, marinara sauce, almond flour, baking powder and Italian seasoning.
3. Add the mixture to the waffle maker.

4. Close the device and cook for minutes.

5. Open it and transfer chaffle to a plate.

6. Let cool for 2 minutes.

7. Repeat the steps with the remaining batter.

8. Top with the grated Parmesan and serve.

Nutrition:

Calories 17 Total Fat 14.3g Saturated Fat 7.5g Cholesterol 118mg Sodium 300mg Potassium 326mg Total Carbohydrate 1.8g Dietary Fiber 0.1g Protein 11.1g Total Sugars 0.4g

Pumpkin-Cinnamon Churro Sticks

Preparation time:

10 minutes

Cooking time:

14 minutes

Servings: 2

Ingredients:

- 3 tbsp coconut flour
- ¼ cup pumpkin puree
- 1 egg, beaten
- ½ cup finely grated mozzarella cheese
- 2 tbsp sugar-free maple syrup + more for serving
- 1 tsp baking powder
- 1 tsp vanilla extract
- ½ tsp pumpkin spice seasoning
- 1/8 tsp salt
- 1 tbsp cinnamon powder

Directions:

1. Preheat the waffle iron.

2. Mix all the Ingredients in a medium bowl until well combined.

3. Open the iron and add half of the mixture. Close and cook until golden brown and crispy, 7 minutes.

4. Remove the chaffle onto a plate and make 1 more with the remaining batter.

5. Cut each chaffle into sticks, drizzle the top with more maple syrup and Servings after.

Nutrition:

Calories 219 Fats 9.72g Carbs 8.64g Net carbs 4.34g Protein 25.27g

Low Carb Keto Broccoli Cheese Waffles

Preparation time:

5 minutes

Cooking time:

5 minutes

Servings: 2

Ingredients:

- 1 cup broccoli, processed
- 1 cup shredded cheddar cheese
- 1/3 cup grated parmesan cheese
- 2 eggs, beats

Directions:

1. spray the Cooking spray on the waffle iron and preheat.
2. Use a powerful blender or food processor to process the broccoli until rice consistency.

3. Mix all Ingredients in a medium bowl.

4. Add 1/3 of the mixture to the waffle iron and cook for 4-5 minutes until golden.

Nutrition:

Calories 160 Total fat 11.8g 18% Cholesterol 121mg 40% Sodium 221.8mg 9% Total carbohydrate 5.1g 2% Dietary fiber 1.7g 7% Sugars 1.2g Protein 10g 20% Vitamin a 133.5 g 9% Vitamin c 7.3mg 12%

Bagel Seasoning Chaffles

Preparation time:

10 minutes

Cooking time:

20 minutes

Servings: 4

Ingredients

- 1 large organic egg
- 1 cup mozzarella cheese, shredded
- 1 tablespoon almond flour
- 1 teaspoon organic baking powder
- 2 teaspoons bagel seasoning
- ¼ teaspoon garlic powder
- ¼ teaspoon onion powder

Directions:

1. Preheat a mini waffle iron and then grease it.
2. In a medium bowl, put all ingredients and with a fork, mix until well combined.

3. Place ¼ of the mixture into preheated waffle iron and cook for about 3–4 minutes.
4. Repeat with the remaining mixture.
5. Serve warm.

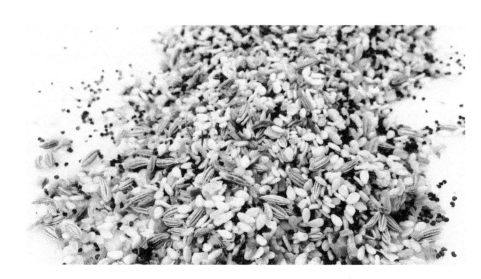

Protein Cheddar Chaffles

Preparation time:

15 minutes

Cooking time:

48 minutes

Servings: 8

Ingredients

- ½ cup golden flax seeds meal
- ½ cup almond flour
- 2 tablespoons unflavored whey protein powder
- 1 teaspoon organic baking powder
- Salt and ground black pepper, to taste
- ¾ cup cheddar cheese, shredded
- 1/3 cup unsweetened almond milk
- 2 tablespoons unsalted butter, melted
- 2 large organic eggs, beaten

Directions:

1. Preheat a mini waffle iron and then grease it.
2. In a large bowl, add flax seeds meal, flour, protein powder, and baking powder, and mix well.
3. Stir in the cheddar cheese.
4. In another bowl, add the remaining ingredients and beat until well combined.
5. Add the egg mixture into the bowl with flax seeds meal mixture and mix until well combined.
6. Place desired amount of the mixture into preheated waffle iron.
7. Cook for about 4–6 minutes.
8. Repeat with the remaining mixture.
9. Serve warm.

Chicken Jalapeño Chaffles

Preparation time:

10 minutes

Cooking time:

10 minutes

Servings: 2

Ingredients:

- ½ cup grass-fed cooked chicken, chopped
- 1 organic egg, beaten
- ¼ cup cheddar cheese, shredded
- 2 tablespoons Parmesan cheese, shredded
- 1 teaspoon cream cheese, softened
- 1 small jalapeño pepper, chopped
- 1/8 teaspoon onion powder
- 1/8 teaspoon garlic powder

Directions:

1. Preheat a mini waffle iron and then grease it.

2. In a medium bowl, put all ingredients and with your hands, mix until well combined.
3. Place half of the mixture into preheated waffle iron and cook for about 4–5 minutes.
4. Repeat with the remaining mixture.
5. Serve warm.

Chicken & Bacon Chaffles

Preparation time:

10 minutes

Cooking time:

8 minutes

Servings: 2

Ingredients

- 1 organic egg, beaten
- 1/3 cup grass-fed cooked chicken, chopped
- 1 cooked bacon slice, crumbled
- 1/3 cup pepper jack cheese, shredded
- 1 teaspoon powdered ranch dressing

Directions:

1. Preheat a mini waffle iron and then grease it.
2. In a medium bowl, put all ingredients and with a fork, mix until well combined.

3. Place half of the mixture into preheated waffle iron and cook for about 3–4 minutes or until golden-brown.
4. Repeat with the remaining mixture.
5. Serve warm.

Sausage Chaffles

Preparation time:

15 minutes

Cooking time:

1 hour

Servings: 12

Ingredients:

- 1 pound gluten-free bulk Italian sausage, crumbled
- 1 organic egg, beaten
- 1 cup sharp cheddar cheese, shredded
- ¼ cup Parmesan cheese, grated
- 1 cup almond flour
- 2 teaspoons organic baking powder

Directions:

1. Preheat a mini waffle iron and then grease it.

2. In a medium bowl, put all ingredients and with your hands, mix until well combined.
3. Place about 3 tablespoons of the mixture into preheated waffle iron and cook for about 3 minutes.
4. Carefully, flip the chaffle and cook for about 2 minutes.
5. Repeat with the remaining mixture.
6. Serve warm.

Sausage & Veggie Chaffles

Preparation time:

15 minutes

Cooking time:

20 minutes

Servings: 4

Ingredients:

- 1/3 cup unsweetened almond milk
- 4 medium organic eggs
- 2 tablespoons gluten-free breakfast sausage, cut into slices
- 2 tablespoons broccoli florets, chopped
- 2 tablespoons bell peppers, seeded and chopped
- 2 tablespoons mozzarella cheese, shredded

Directions:

1. Preheat a waffle iron and then grease it.

2. In a medium bowl, add the almond milk and eggs and beat well.
3. Place the remaining ingredients and stir to combine well.
4. Place desired amount of the mixture into preheated waffle iron.
5. Cook for about 5 minutes.
6. Repeat with the remaining mixture.
7. Serve warm.

Cauliflower & Chives Chaffles

Preparation time:

15 minutes

Cooking time:

1 hour 4 minutes

Servings: 8

Ingredients:

- 1½ cups cauliflower, grated
- ½ cup cheddar cheese, shredded
- ½ cup mozzarella cheese, shredded
- ¼ cup Parmesan cheese, shredded
- 3 large organic eggs, beaten
- 3 tablespoons fresh chives, chopped
- ¼ teaspoon red pepper flakes, crushed
- Salt and ground black pepper, to taste

Directions:

1. Preheat a mini waffle iron and then grease it.

2. In a food processor, place all the ingredients and pulse until well combined.

3. Divide the mixture into 8 portions.

4. Place 1 portion of the mixture into preheated waffle iron and cook for about 8 minutes.

5. Repeat with the remaining mixture.

6. Serve warm.

Spinach Chaffles

Preparation time:

15 minutes

Cooking time:

20 minutes

Servings: 4

Ingredients:

- 1 large organic egg, beaten
- 1 cup ricotta cheese, crumbled
- ½ cup mozzarella cheese, shredded
- ¼ cup Parmesan cheese, grated
- 4 ounces frozen spinach, thawed and squeezed
- 1 garlic clove, minced
- Salt and ground black pepper, to taste

Directions:

1. Preheat a mini waffle iron and then grease it.

2. In a medium bowl, put all ingredients and with a fork, mix until well combined.
3. Place ¼ of the mixture into preheated waffle iron and cook for about 4–5 minutes.
4. Repeat with the remaining mixture.
5. Serve warm.

Zucchini Chaffles

Preparation time:

10 minutes

Cooking time:

10 minutes

Servings: 2

Ingredients:

- 1 organic egg, beaten
- ¼ cup mozzarella cheese, shredded
- 2 tablespoons Parmesan cheese, grated
- ½ of small zucchini, grated and squeezed
- ¼ teaspoon dried basil, crushed
- Freshly ground black pepper, to taste

Directions:

1. Preheat a mini waffle iron and then grease it.
2. In a medium bowl, put all ingredients and with a fork, mix until well combined.

3. Place half of the mixture into preheated waffle iron and cook for about 4–5 minutes.
4. Repeat with the remaining mixture.
5. Serve warm.

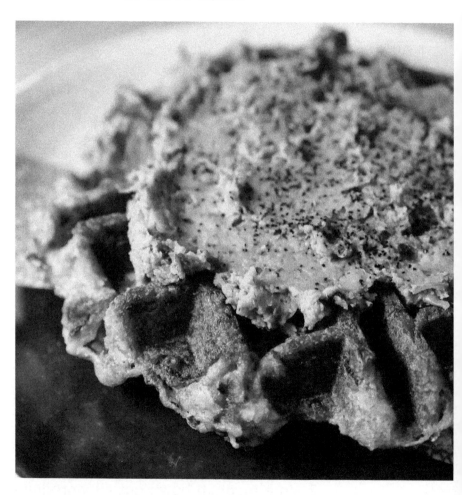

Chicken Chaffles

Preparation time:

10 minutes

Cooking time:

8 minutes

Servings: 2

Ingredients:

- 1 1/3 cups grass-fed cooked chicken, chopped
- ½ cup cheddar cheese, shredded
- 1 tablespoon sugar-free BBQ sauce
- 1 organic egg, beaten
- 1 tablespoon almond flour

Directions:

1. Preheat a mini waffle iron and then grease it.
2. In a bowl, put all ingredients and with your hands, mix until well combined.

3. Place half of the mixture into preheated waffle iron and cook for about 4 minutes.

4. Repeat with the remaining mixture.

5. Serve warm.

Herb Chaffles

Preparation time:

15 minutes

Cooking time:

12 minutes

Servings: 4

Ingredients:

- 4 tablespoons almond flour
- 1 tablespoon coconut flour
- 1 teaspoon mixed dried herbs
- ½ teaspoon organic baking powder
- ¼ teaspoon garlic powder
- ¼ teaspoon onion powder
- Salt and ground black pepper, to taste
- ¼ cup cream cheese, softened
- 3 large organic eggs
- ½ cup cheddar cheese, grated
- 1/3 cup Parmesan cheese, grated

Directions:

1. Preheat a waffle iron and then grease it.

2. In a bowl, mix together the flours, dried herbs, baking powder, and seasoning, and mix well.

3. In a separate bowl, put cream cheese and eggs and beat until well combined.

4. Add the flour mixture, cheddar, and Parmesan cheese, and mix until well combined.

5. Place the desired amount of the mixture into preheated waffle iron and cook for about 2–3 minutes.

6. Repeat with the remaining mixture.

7. Serve warm.

Cauliflower Chaffles

Preparation time:

15 minutes

Cooking time:

32 minutes

Servings: 4

Ingredients:

- 1½ cups cauliflower, grated
- ½ cup cheddar cheese
- ½ cup mozzarella cheese
- ¼ cup Parmesan cheese
- 3 large organic eggs
- 3 tablespoons fresh chives, chopped
- ¼ teaspoon red pepper flakes, crushed
- Salt and ground black pepper, to taste

Directions:

1. Preheat a waffle iron and then grease it.

2. In a food processor, place all the ingredients and pulse until well combined.
3. Place the desired amount of the mixture into preheated waffle iron and cook for about 7–8 minutes.
4. Repeat with the remaining mixture.
5. Serve warm.

Jalapeño Chaffles

Preparation time:

5 minutes

Cooking time:

10 minutes

Serving: 2

Ingredients:

- 1 organic egg, beaten
- ½ cup cheddar cheese, shredded
- ½ tablespoon jalapeño pepper, chopped

Directions:

1. Preheat a mini waffle iron and then grease it.
2. In a medium bowl, put all ingredients and with a fork, mix until well combined.
3. Place half of the mixture into preheated waffle iron and cook for about 3–5 minutes.

4. Repeat with the remaining mixture.

5. Serve warm.

Scallion Chaffles

Preparation time:

10 minutes

Cooking time:

8 minutes

Servings: 2

Ingredients:

- 1 organic egg, beaten
- ½ cup mozzarella cheese, shredded
- 1 tablespoon scallion, chopped
- ½ teaspoon Italian seasoning

Directions:

1. Preheat a mini waffle iron and then grease it.
2. In a medium bowl, put all ingredients and with a fork, mix until well combined.
3. Place half of the mixture into preheated waffle iron and cook for about 4 minutes.

4. Repeat with the remaining mixture.

5. Serve warm.

Broccoli Chaffles

Preparation time:

10 minutes

Cooking time:

8 minutes

Servings: 2

Ingredients:

- 1 organic egg, beaten
- ½ cup cheddar cheese, shredded
- ¼ cup fresh broccoli, chopped
- 1 tablespoon almond flour
- ¼ teaspoon garlic powder

Directions:

1. Preheat a mini waffle iron and then grease it.
2. In a bowl, put all ingredients and mix until well combined.
3. Place half of the mixture into preheated waffle iron and cook for about 4 minutes.

4. Repeat with the remaining mixture.

5. Serve warm.

Hot Sauce Jalapeño Chaffles

Preparation time:

10 minutes

Cooking time:

8 minutes

Servings: 2

Ingredients:

- ½ cup plus 2 teaspoons cheddar cheese, shredded and divided
- 1 organic egg, beaten
- 6 jalapeño pepper slices
- ¼ teaspoon hot sauce
- Pinch of salt

Directions:

1. Preheat a mini waffle iron and then grease it.
2. In a bowl, add ½ cup of cheese and remaining ingredients and mix until well combined.

3. Place about 1 teaspoon of cheese in the bottom of the waffle maker for about 30 seconds before adding the mixture

4. Place half of the mixture into preheated waffle iron and cook for about 3–4 minutes.

5. Repeat with the remaining cheese and mixture.

6. Serve warm.

BBQ Rub Chaffles

Preparation time:

5 minutes

Cooking time:

20 minutes

Servings: 4

Ingredients:

- 2 organic eggs, beaten
- 1 cup cheddar cheese, shredded
- ½ teaspoon BBQ rub
- ¼ teaspoon organic baking powder

Directions:

1. Preheat a mini waffle iron and then grease it.
2. In a medium bowl, put all ingredients and with a fork, mix until well combined.
3. Place ¼ of the mixture into preheated waffle iron and cook for about 5 minutes.

4. Repeat with the remaining mixture.

5. Serve warm.

Easy Breakfast Chaffle

Preparation time:

10 minutes

Cooking time:

5 minutes

Serving: 2

Ingredients:

- 1 egg, lightly beaten
- 1/2 cup mozzarella cheese, shredded

Directions:

1. Preheat your mini waffle maker.
2. In a bowl, mix egg and shredded cheese until combined.
3. Pour half of the batter in the hot waffle maker and cook until golden brown. Repeat with the remaining batter.
4. Serve and enjoy.

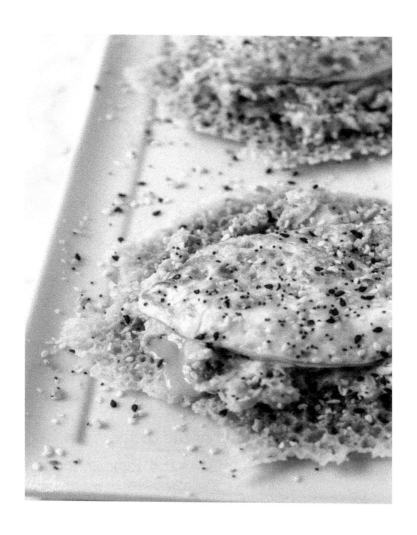

Tuna Chaffle

Preparation time:

15 minutes

Cooking time:

10 minutes

Servings: 2

Ingredients:

- 1 egg, lightly beaten
- 1/2 cup cheddar cheese, shredded
- tuna, drained
- Pinch of salt

Directions:

1. Preheat your waffle maker.
2. In a small bowl, mix egg, cheese, tuna, and salt until combined.
3. Pour half of the batter in the hot waffle maker and cook for 4 minutes or until golden brown. Repeat with the remaining batter.
4. Serve and enjoy.

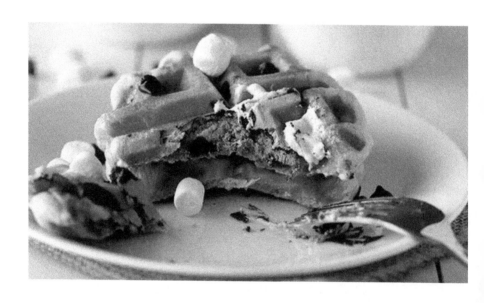

Delicious Garlic Chaffle

Preparation time:

20 minutes

Cooking time:

10 minutes

Servings: 2

Ingredients:

- 1 egg
- 1 tsp coconut flour
- 1 tbsp parmesan cheese, grated
- 1/2 cup cheddar cheese, shredded
- 1/4 tsp baking powder
- 1/2 cup mozzarella cheese, shredded
- 1/4 tsp garlic powder
- 1 tbsp butter, melted
- Pinch of salt

Directions:

1. Preheat the waffle maker.
2. In a small bowl, mix egg, cheddar cheese, parmesan cheese, coconut

flour, baking powder, and salt until well combined.

3. Spray waffle maker with cooking spray.

4. Pour half of the batter in the hot waffle maker and cook for 4 minutes or until golden brown. Repeat with the remaining batter.

5. In a small bowl, mix butter and garlic powder.

6. Brush chaffles with butter garlic mixture and top with mozzarella cheese.

7. Broil chaffles until cheese melted.

8. Serve and enjoy.

Bacon Chaffle

Preparation time:

20 minutes

Cooking time:

10 minutes

Servings: 6

Ingredients:

- 1 egg, lightly beaten
- 1/2 tsp baking powder, gluten-free
- 1/2 tsp dried parsley
- 1/4 tsp onion powder
- 1/4 tsp garlic powder
- 1/4 tsp Swerve
- 1 cup cheddar cheese, shredded
- 1 1/2 tbsp butter, melted
- 4 bacon slices, cooked and crumbled
- 1/4 cup sour cream
- 1/2 cup almond flour

Directions:

1. Preheat your mini waffle maker.

2. In a bowl, mix almond flour, garlic powder, onion powder, and baking powder until combined.

3. In another bowl, add egg, cheese, butter, bacon, parsley, sour cream, and bacon and mix until combined.

4. Add almond flour mixture into the egg mixture and mix well.

5. Pour 2-3 tablespoons of batter in the hot waffle maker and cook for 5-6 minutes or until golden brown.

6. Repeat with the remaining batter.

7. Serve and enjoy.

Savoury Cheddar Cheese Chaffle

Preparation time:

10 minutes

Cooking time:

5 minutes

Servings: 1

Ingredients:

- 1 egg
- 1/4 tsp garlic powder
- 1/4 tsp onion powder
- 1/4 tsp baking powder, gluten-free
- 2 tbsp almond flour
- 1/4 cup cheddar cheese, shredded
- Pinch of salt

Directions:

1. Preheat your waffle maker.
2. In a bowl, whisk together egg, garlic powder, baking powder, onion powder, almond flour, cheese, and salt.

3. Spray waffle maker with cooking spray.
4. Pour batter in the hot waffle maker and cook for 3-5 minutes or until set.
5. Serve and enjoy.

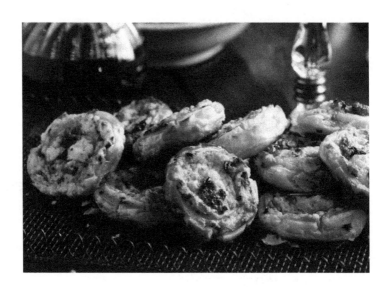

Perfect Jalapeno Chaffle

Preparation time:

15 minutes

Cooking time:

10 minutes

Servings: 6

Ingredients:

- 3 eggs
- 1 cup cheddar cheese, shredded
- 8 oz cream cheese
- 2 jalapeno peppers, diced
- 4 bacon slices, cooked and crumbled
- 1/2 tsp baking powder
- 3 tbsp coconut flour
- 1/4 tsp sea salt

Directions:

1. Preheat your waffle maker.
2. In a small bowl, mix coconut flour, baking powder, and salt.

3. In a medium bowl, beat cream cheese using a hand mixer until fluffy.

4. In a large bowl, beat eggs until fluffy.

5. Add cheddar cheese and half cup cream in eggs and beat until well combined.

6. Add coconut flour mixture to egg mixture and mix until combined.

7. Add jalapeno pepper and stir well.

8. Spray waffle maker with cooking spray.

9. Pour 1/4 cup batter in the hot waffle maker and cook for 4-5 minutes. Repeat with the remaining batter. Once chaffle is slightly cool then top with remaining cream cheese and bacon.

10. Serve and enjoy.

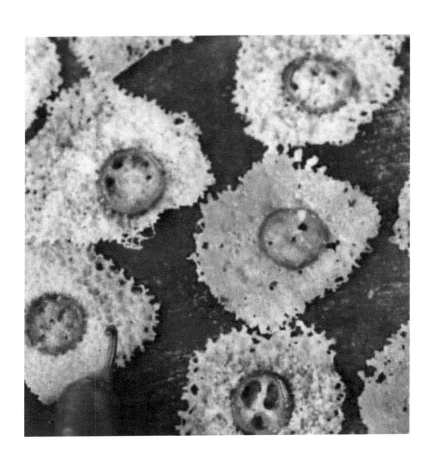

Crunchy Zucchini Chaffle

Preparation time:

15 minutes

Cooking time:

10 minutes

Servings: 8

Ingredients:

- 2 eggs, lightly beaten
- 1 garlic clove, minced
- 1 1/2 tbsp onion, minced
- 1 cup cheddar cheese, grated
- 1 small zucchini, grated and squeeze out all liquid

Directions:

1. Preheat your waffle maker.
2. In a bowl, mix eggs, garlic, onion, zucchini, and cheese until well combined.
3. Spray waffle maker with cooking spray.

4. Pour 1/4 cup batter in the hot waffle maker and cook for 5 minutes or until golden brown.

5. Repeat with the remaining batter.

6. Serve and enjoy.

Simple Cheese Bacon Chaffles

Preparation time:

10 minutes

Cooking time:

10 minutes

Servings: 4

Ingredients:

- 2 eggs, lightly beaten
- 1/4 tsp garlic powder
- 2 bacon slices, cooked and chopped
- 3/4 cup cheddar cheese, shredded

Directions:

1. Preheat your mini waffle maker and spray with cooking spray.
2. In a bowl, mix eggs, garlic powder, bacon, and cheese.
3. Pour 2 tbsp of the batter in the hot waffle maker and cook for 2-3 minutes or until set. Repeat with the remaining batter.

4. Serve and enjoy.

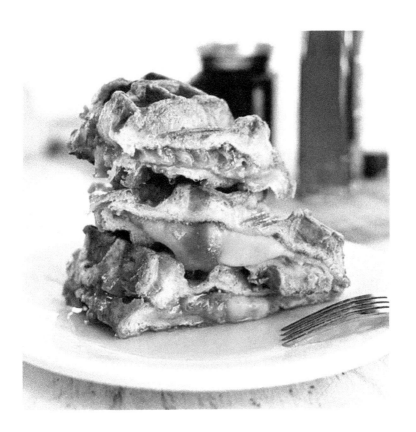

Cheddar Cauliflower Chaffle

Preparation time:

10 minutes

Cooking time:

5 minutes

Servings: 1

Ingredients:

- 1 egg, lightly beaten
- 1 tbsp almond flour
- 1/4 cup cheddar cheese, shredded
- 1/2 cup cauliflower rice
- Pepper
- Salt

Directions:

1. Preheat your waffle maker.
2. Add all ingredients into the bowl and mix until well combined.
3. Spray waffle maker with cooking spray.

4. Pour batter in the hot waffle maker and cook for 8 minutes or until golden brown.

5. Serve and enjoy.

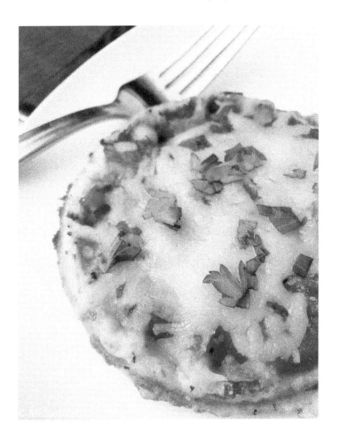

Perfect Keto Chaffle

Preparation time:

10 minutes

Cooking time:

8 minutes

Servings: 2

Ingredients:

- 2 eggs, lightly beaten
- 1/2 cup mozzarella cheese, shredded
- 1/2 cup cheddar cheese, shredded
- 1/4 tsp baking powder, gluten-free
- 1 tbsp almond flour
- 1/4 tsp cinnamon
- 1/4 tsp red chili flakes
- 1/4 tsp salt

Directions:

1. Preheat your waffle maker and spray with cooking spray.
2. In a bowl, whisk eggs with baking powder, almond flour, and salt.

3. Add remaining ingredients and mix until well combined.

4. Pour half of the batter in the hot waffle maker and cook for 3-5 minutes or until golden brown. Repeat with the remaining batter.

5. Serve and enjoy.

Cabbage Chaffle

Preparation time:

15 minutes

Cooking time:

5 minutes

Servings: 2

Ingredients:

- 1 egg, lightly beaten
- 1/3 cup mozzarella cheese, grated
- ½ bacon slice, chopped
- 1 ½ tbsp green onion, sliced
- 2 tbsp cabbage, chopped
- 2 tbsp almond flour
- Pepper
- Salt

Directions:

1. Add all ingredients in a bowl and stir to combine.
2. Spray waffle maker with cooking spray.

3. Pour half of the batter in the hot waffle maker and cook until golden brown.
4. Repeat with the remaining batter.
5. Serve and enjoy.

Simple Ham Chaffle

Preparation time:

10 minutes

Cooking time:

8 minutes

Servings: 2

Ingredients:

- 1 egg, lightly beaten
- 1/4 cup ham, chopped
- 1/2 cup cheddar cheese, shredded
- 1/4 tsp garlic salt
- For Dip:
- 1 1/2 tsp Dijon mustard
- 1 tbsp mayonnaise

Directions:

1. Preheat your waffle maker.
2. Whisk eggs in a bowl.
3. Stir in ham, cheese, and garlic salt until combine.

4. Spray waffle maker with cooking spray.
5. Pour half of the batter in the hot waffle maker and cook for 3-4 minutes or until golden brown.
6. Repeat with the remaining batter.
7. For Dip: In a small bowl, mix mustard and mayonnaise.
8. Serve chaffle with dip.

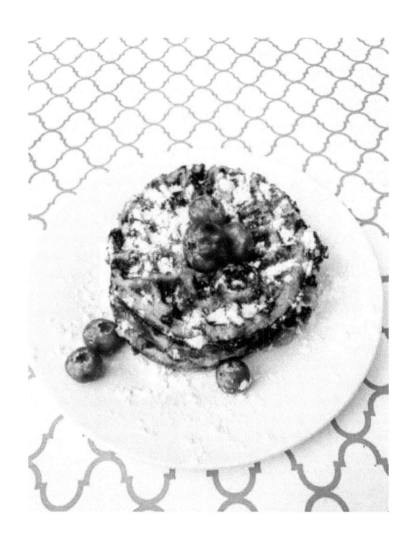